ECZEMA ELEVATION

Holistic Therapies For Soothing Skin Conditions

Find Relief From Eczema And Other Skin Conditions Through A Holistic Approach To Skincare And Innovative Therapeutic Solutions

DR. BRIDGET PROMISE

Table of Contents

CHAPTER ONE 4

Introduction 4

Understanding Eczema: Unraveling The Skin Condition 5

The Effects Of Eczema On Daily 6

Conventional Treatments And 8

CHAPTER TWO 14

Accepting Holistic Approaches To...............14

Mind-Body Connection: Stress 15

Nourishing Your Skin From The...................17

Essential Skincare Habits For 19

Natural Treatments & Herbs For 24

CHAPTER THREE 31

Mindful Living: Incorporating.....................31

Environmental Considerations:...................34

The Role Of Allergens And Irritants In Eczema Flare-Ups...39

CHAPTER FOUR 42

Structure A Helpful Set Of Connections: The Significance Of Community.........................42

CHAPTER FIVE 45

Maintaining Eczema Elevation: 45

Conclusion: Your Journey To Soothe And
Elevate Your Skin 49

CHAPTER ONE

Introduction

Eczema is a persistent skin disorder that causes inflammation, redness, and itching in millions of individuals worldwide. While the word "eczema" is often used to describe a variety of skin disorders, the most prevalent is atopic dermatitis.

This inflammatory illness may appear at any age, however, it is most common during infancy. Understanding the subtleties of eczema is critical for people dealing with its consequences daily. In this examination, we'll look at the complexities of eczema, its influence on everyday living, and the limits of traditional therapies.

Understanding Eczema: Unraveling The Skin Condition

Eczema is a complex skin illness that causes more than just physical pain. It's a complicated interaction of genetic, environmental, and immune system elements.

While the specific origin is unknown, experts think that a mix of genetic predisposition and environmental stimuli contribute to the development of eczema.

Genetics plays an important role since those who have a family history of allergic disorders like asthma or hay fever are more prone to develop eczema.

The immune system's reaction to specific irritants or allergens causes inflammation in the skin, resulting in the classic symptoms of eczema: redness, itching, and the creation of rash-like areas.

The Effects Of Eczema On Daily Life

Living with eczema goes much beyond the apparent signs on the skin. Constant itching, pain, and the psychological toll may have a substantial influence on a person's quality of life. The persistent urge to avoid scratching, particularly during flare-ups, turns into a daily fight. Eczema often causes sleep disruptions because itching worsens at night, interfering with comfortable sleep.

Furthermore, the apparent form of eczema may cause social and emotional difficulties. Eczema sufferers may feel self-conscious, embarrassed, or isolated. The unpredictability of flare-ups, along with the condition's apparent character, may lead to a loss of self-esteem and confidence.

Children with eczema may experience extra challenges since the illness may disrupt their everyday activities and social relationships. Eczema's pain and visibility may lead to taunting or bullying, which may have a negative influence on a child's mental health and social development.

Conventional Treatments And Limitations

Conventional therapies for eczema concentrate largely on symptom relief and flare-up management. Emollients, topical corticosteroids, and antihistamines are widely given to relieve itching, decrease inflammation, and enhance general skin health. While these therapies may give temporary comfort, they often have restrictions.

First, the efficacy of traditional therapy differs from person to person. This unpredictability emphasizes the necessity for a tailored approach to eczema treatment.

Second, long-term usage of some drugs, such as topical

corticosteroids, may have dangers. Prolonged use might cause skin thinning, discoloration, and other negative effects. This entails striking a delicate balance between treating symptoms and reducing possible side effects.

Furthermore, traditional therapies typically fail to address the underlying causes of eczema. While they may give comfort during flare-ups, they may not prevent symptoms from recurring. This emphasizes the need to use a comprehensive strategy that takes into account lifestyle variables, environmental triggers, and general immune system health.

In recent years, there has been a surge of interest in complementary and alternative therapy for eczema. These techniques often concentrate on correcting underlying imbalances in the body, encouraging skin health from within, and avoiding the need for long-term medicine. Individuals seeking a more complete and sustainable approach to eczema are exploring alternatives such as dietary changes, probiotics, and natural therapies.

Eczema, with its complex interplay of genetic, environmental, and immunological variables, presents a tremendous challenge to individuals afflicted. The influence on everyday living goes beyond physical symptoms to include emotional well-being and social relationships. Conventional therapies, although giving comfort, have limits and may not be a long-term solution.

As we continue to understand the complexity of eczema, a comprehensive strategy that takes into account each individual's specific circumstances becomes more vital. Exploring alternative therapy and making lifestyle changes might pave the door for a more complete and individualized approach to eczema care. Understanding the problem and its implications is the first step toward comprehensive well-being on the path to successful eczema therapy.

CHAPTER TWO
Accepting Holistic Approaches To Eczema Relief

Living with eczema may be difficult since this chronic skin disease frequently requires a diverse strategy for successful treatment.

While topical treatments are routinely recommended, adopting holistic techniques that address the mind-body connection, feed the skin from within, and instill fundamental hygiene habits may help manage and alleviate eczema symptoms.

Mind-Body Connection: Stress Management For Skin Wellness.

Eczema treatment relies heavily on the complex link between the mind and the body. Stress, a well-known cause of eczema flare-ups, may worsen symptoms and slow the healing process. As a result, integrating stress management practices is critical for improving general skin health.

Mindfulness methods, such as meditation and deep breathing exercises, have shown potential in lowering stress and, as a result, relieving eczema symptoms. These strategies encourage relaxation, so breaking the stress-induced loop that often exacerbates skin issues. Furthermore, exercises such as yoga and tai chi not only help the body but also the mind, promoting a holistic approach to eczema management.

Cognitive-behavioral therapy (CBT) is another effective method for treating the mind-body link in eczema treatment. This therapy method assists patients in identifying and changing negative thinking patterns and actions that might lead to stress and worsen skin issues. CBT helps people manage the emotional elements of living with eczema by fostering a positive outlook and giving coping techniques.

Nourishing Your Skin From The Inside Out: Dietary Strategies

The proverb "you are what you eat" is especially relevant when it comes to eczema management. A well-balanced and healthy diet may improve skin health by alleviating symptoms and promoting internal healing.

Incorporating anti-inflammatory ingredients into your diet may be life-changing for eczema patients. Omega-3 fatty acids, found in fatty fish, flaxseeds, and walnuts, are anti-inflammatory and may help decrease skin irritation and itching. Similarly, eating antioxidant-rich foods like berries, leafy greens, and green tea might help the body's natural defenses against oxidative stress and inflammation.

Identifying and avoiding possible trigger foods is another critical component of a comprehensive dietary approach to eczema management. Dairy, gluten, and preservatives are common trigger foods. Keeping a food diary and talking with a healthcare expert or qualified dietitian may assist in identifying particular triggers and offer personalized dietary recommendations.

Hydration is essential for skin health, and those who have eczema should drink enough water. Staying hydrated helps the skin's barrier function by minimizing excessive dryness and creating a stronger skin barrier. Herbal teas, as well as water-rich fruits and vegetables, may help to maintain general hydration.

Essential Skincare Habits For Eczema Sufferers

Aside from reducing stress and eating a skin-friendly diet,

developing important skincare practices is critical for controlling eczema and improving skin health. These routines are aimed at strengthening the skin's natural barrier, reducing irritation, and improving moisture retention.

Choosing the appropriate skincare products is an important first step. Choose fragrance-free and hypoallergenic products to reduce the chance of skin irritation. To keep skin hydrated, use moisturizers formulated particularly for sensitive skin frequently. Emollients, which retain moisture, and humectants, which draw moisture to the skin, may be very effective.

When bathing, use lukewarm water and gentle, fragrance-free cleansers. Hot water may deplete the skin's natural oils, aggravating dryness and irritation. Patting the skin dry with a soft towel and immediately applying moisturizer may help retain moisture and avoid overdrying.

Wearing loose, airy textiles like cotton may help prevent skin friction and discomfort. Avoiding tight garments and abrasive textiles that might aggravate eczema symptoms is a simple but useful practice for improving skin comfort.

Understanding individual triggers is essential for efficient eczema therapy. Identifying and reducing exposure to triggers, such as certain materials, skincare components, or environmental variables, may greatly decrease the frequency and severity of eczema flare-ups.

To summarize, adopting holistic methods for eczema treatment includes acknowledging the interdependence of the mind and body, feeding the skin from the inside with a balanced diet, and developing key skincare practices. By addressing the underlying causes and triggers of eczema, people may make proactive efforts to manage symptoms and achieve long-term skin health. A holistic approach not only focuses on symptom treatment but also teaches people how to live a healthy lifestyle that improves general well-being and resilience in the face of eczema issues.

Eczema is a persistent skin disorder marked by inflammation, redness, itching, and, in rare cases, blisters. While traditional medical treatments exist, a growing number of people are turning to natural remedies and alternative therapies to control and relieve their eczema symptoms. In this inquiry, we will look at natural cures such as herbs, alternative therapies such as acupuncture and acupressure, the advantages of mindful living via meditation and relaxation methods, and how to create an eczema-friendly house.

Natural Treatments & Herbs For Eczema

Many people look for natural remedies and herbal therapies to help them manage their eczema. Nature has offered a variety of herbs with anti-inflammatory, antibacterial, and calming characteristics that may help treat eczema symptoms.

Calendula is a regularly used plant. Calendula, often known as marigold, has anti-inflammatory and antibacterial characteristics that may help lessen the redness and irritation caused by eczema. To provide relief, use calendula oil or cream topically to the afflicted regions.

Chamomile is another plant that has calming characteristics and may help eczema patients. Chamomile, whether taken as a tea or applied topically, helps soothe sensitive skin and encourage healing. Its anti-inflammatory and anti-itch characteristics make it a popular option among people looking for natural remedies.

The aloe vera plant, known for its therapeutic powers, is also often used to treat eczema. When applied to damaged regions, aloe vera gel moisturizes the skin, reduces inflammation, and speeds up the healing process. Its cooling effect gives quick relief from itching and pain.

Evening primrose oil, which contains gamma-linolenic acid (GLA), is recognized for its anti-inflammatory properties. Evening primrose oil, taken as a supplement, may help treat eczema symptoms by reducing internal inflammation.

These natural solutions frequently work best when taken regularly over time, either in conjunction with conventional treatments or as solo choices for people seeking a holistic approach to eczema care.

Exploring Alternative Therapies: Acupuncture and Acupressure.

Acupuncture and acupressure, ancient Chinese medicinal treatments, are gaining popularity for their ability to treat eczema symptoms. These treatments are based on the notion that the body's essential energy, or qi, runs along particular paths known as meridians. Acupoints along these meridians may be stimulated to restore balance and harmony in the body.

Acupuncture is the process of inserting tiny needles into particular acupoints to stimulate the passage of qi and facilitate healing. According to several studies, acupuncture may help lessen the itching and inflammation associated with eczema. The specific method by which acupuncture exerts its benefits on eczema is not entirely known, however, it is thought to entail the control of immunological responses and the production of anti-inflammatory chemicals.

Acupressure, a non-invasive alternative to acupuncture, involves applying pressure to acupoints using fingers, palms, or specialized equipment. It is considered to offer comparable advantages in terms of improving energy flow and resolving imbalances that lead to eczema symptoms.

While research on acupuncture and acupressure for eczema is still growing, some patients report beneficial benefits, including decreased irritation and general improvement in skin condition.

As with any alternative treatment, it's crucial to contact with a skilled practitioner to verify its compatibility and discuss how it might be incorporated into an individual's overall eczema care strategy.

CHAPTER THREE

Mindful Living: Incorporating Meditation And Relaxation Techniques

Stress is a well-known cause of eczema flare-ups, and adopting mindful living techniques may be an effective method to manage stress and its effects on the skin.

Meditation, a technique that includes concentrating the mind and relaxing the thoughts, has shown promise in lowering stress and boosting general well-being.

Mindfulness meditation, in particular, teaches people to be

present in the moment, observing thoughts and feelings without judgment. This heightened awareness may help stop the cycle of stress and worry that frequently exacerbates eczema symptoms. Regular mindfulness meditation practice has been connected with lower inflammation and better skin conditions in some patients with eczema.

In addition to meditation, relaxation methods such as deep breathing exercises and progressive muscular relaxation might be effective. These techniques assist in stimulating the body's relaxation response, counteracting the stress-induced inflammation that may lead to eczema flares.

Incorporating mindfulness into everyday life extends beyond formal meditation sessions. It entails being present throughout ordinary tasks, relishing the sensory sensations, and reducing multitasking. By practicing mindfulness, persons with eczema may establish a more resilient attitude and perhaps lower the frequency and severity of flare-ups.

Environmental Considerations: Creating An Eczema-Friendly Home

Beyond herbal medicines and alternative therapies, the environment in which persons with eczema live may dramatically affect their skin health. Creating an eczema-friendly home entails making smart decisions that limit possible irritants and allergies.

Choosing hypoallergenic bedding and clothes helps prevent skin irritation. Fabrics like cotton and silk are breathable and less prone to generate friction or retain moisture against the skin. Washing bedding and clothes using fragrance-free, hypoallergenic detergents further decreases the chance of skin discomfort.

Maintaining a stable and pleasant room temperature is vital for those with eczema. Extreme conditions, whether hot or cold, may provoke flare-ups. Using a humidifier in dry areas may help keep the skin moisturized, avoiding excessive dryness that may worsen eczema symptoms.

Avoiding strong soaps and opting for mild, fragrance-free cleansers helps avoid skin irritation. Moisturizing consistently, particularly after bathing, helps lock in moisture and preserve skin barrier function. Natural moisturizers like coconut oil or shea butter are popular alternatives for their soothing effects.

Consideration should also be paid to possible allergies inside the house. Identifying and reducing exposure to common allergens like dust mites, pet dander, and specific foods may aid in overall eczema control.

In conclusion, investigating natural cures, alternative therapies, adopting mindful living habits, and building an eczema-friendly environment are holistic methods that may complement traditional therapy.

It's crucial to approach eczema treatment with a customized viewpoint, realizing that what helps one person may vary from another. Integrating these factors into a complete eczema care plan may give patients with a more holistic and tailored approach to controlling their disease. As usual, working with healthcare specialists, especially dermatologists and skilled practitioners of alternative medicines, may help people navigate and adjust their eczema management techniques efficiently.

Living with eczema may be tough since the illness generally includes periods of quiet broken by severe flare-ups. One key factor that patients with eczema need to grasp is the involvement of allergens and irritants in initiating these flare-ups.

Additionally, developing a supporting network becomes crucial in overcoming the mental and physical obstacles that come with controlling eczema. In this process, establishing long-term tactics to sustain eczema elevation becomes crucial to attaining persistent relief.

The Role Of Allergens And Irritants In Eczema Flare-Ups

Eczema, also known as atopic dermatitis, is a persistent skin disorder marked by inflammation, itching, and redness. Understanding the elements that lead to flare-ups is critical for optimal treatment. Allergens and irritants have a vital role in initiating these episodes.

Allergens are chemicals that the immune system recognizes as hazardous, resulting in an allergic response. In eczema, typical allergens include pet dander, pollen, mold, and certain foods. Exposure to certain allergens might worsen symptoms and induce flare-ups.

Irritants, on the other hand, are compounds that cause direct irritation to the skin, resulting in inflammation and pain. Harsh soaps, detergents, scents, and even certain textiles may irritate those who have eczema. Identifying and avoiding these triggers is critical for preventing flare-ups and preserving skin health.

Individuals with eczema should attempt to establish an allergen- and irritant-free environment. Making deliberate decisions in everyday life, such as using mild, fragrance-free skin care products, choosing hypoallergenic materials, and cleaning living areas regularly, may help decrease dust and mold.

Regular consultations with a healthcare expert or allergist may help discover particular allergies via testing.

CHAPTER FOUR

Structure A Helpful Set Of Connections: The Significance Of Community

Eczema is more than simply a physical difficulty; it also has an emotional impact. Persistent itching, pain, and visual signs may influence a person's mental health. Building a supporting network is very useful in this situation.

Individuals with eczema rely heavily on their family, friends, and support networks for emotional stability. Loved ones' compassion and sensitivity may make a major difference in dealing with the emotional components of the disease. Joining eczema support groups, whether in person or online, provides a chance to interact with people who have had similar experiences. These forums provide a forum for discussing coping skills, success stories, and empathic understanding.

Furthermore, consulting with healthcare experts, such as dermatologists and mental health specialists, helps to build a complete support system. Dermatologists may give personalized treatment plans and advice, whilst mental health practitioners can provide coping skills for dealing with the emotional effect of living with a chronic disease.

Individuals with eczema must freely speak with their support network about their needs and concerns. Individuals who create a supportive atmosphere may better handle the ups and downs of eczema management, thereby improving their general well-being.

CHAPTER FIVE

Maintaining Eczema Elevation: Long-Term Strategies

While avoiding daily irritants and establishing a strong support network are critical measures, long-term tactics are also essential for sustaining eczema elevation. These techniques emphasize lifestyle changes and preventive actions to avoid flare-ups and improve general skin health.

1. Establishing a Consistent Skincare regimen: Effective eczema treatment requires a gentle and consistent skincare regimen. Using fragrance-free

moisturizers and gentle cleansers helps to keep the skin hydrated and avoid dryness, which is a typical cause of flare-ups.

2. Choosing comfortable clothing may have a big influence on eczema. Choose loose-fitting, breathable textiles like cotton to prevent irritation and enable the skin to breathe. Avoiding rough or scratchy fabrics is critical for preventing friction-related flare-ups.

3. Dietary Modifications: Some foods may trigger eczema flare-ups. Working with a healthcare expert to identify and remove

possible trigger foods may help. Furthermore, eating a well-balanced diet rich in anti-inflammatory foods may improve general skin health.

4. Stress Management: Stress has been linked to eczema flare-ups. Adopting stress-reduction methods like as mindfulness, yoga, or meditation may help to maintain eczema elevation. These routines promote both mental and skin health.

5. Schedule regular follow-ups with healthcare professionals. Consistent contact with healthcare specialists, such as dermatologists

and allergists, is vital. Regular check-ups allow for adjustments to treatment regimens depending on the individual's changing requirements. This preventative strategy may assist in avoiding any flare-ups.

6. Environmental considerations. Eczema management relies heavily on environmental considerations. Maintaining a cool and humid living environment may help avoid excessive dryness, and utilizing air purifiers can help decrease exposure to harmful allergens.

Conclusion: Your Journey To Soothe And Elevate Your Skin

To summarize, controlling eczema is a comprehensive process that includes recognizing and reducing the effect of allergens and irritants, developing a strong support network, and implementing long-term measures for continuous relief.

Individuals with eczema may manage their path with resilience by recognizing and avoiding irritants, cultivating a supportive group, and making proactive lifestyle changes. Remember that every step you take to better understand and manage eczema puts you closer to living a more comfortable and peaceful life.